Psoriatic Arthritis Explained

Understanding Psoriatic Arthritis

Causes, Symptoms, Treatments, Self – Help Techniques, Natural Remedies and Many More!

By Frederick Earlstein

Foreword

Are you suffering from swollen joints, painful muscles, scaly skin patches and flaky scalp? This inflammation is a kind of arthritis that affects a number of people who already have psoriasis. It is called *psoriatic arthritis*. This condition can be quite debilitating as it affects different parts of the body—from the fingertips to the spine—and the illness can range from mild to severe. At present, there is no specific cure for psoriatic arthritis but you can manage the symptoms and prevent further damage to your joints. When there is no treatment or intervention done, both psoriasis and psoriatic arthritis can worsen.

While there is a growing recognition on the pervasiveness of psoriatic arthritis worldwide, not everyone is well-informed and many people are either under-diagnosed or misdiagnosed. Psoriatic arthritis is one of the most prevalent autoimmune diseases worldwide. If you have been diagnosed with psoriatic arthritis, the best thing you can do is to educate yourself about it.

In this book, you will learn about the symptoms of the ailment, treatment and management options, how changing your diet can improve your condition, and how you can be in control of your life.

Table of Contents

Introduction

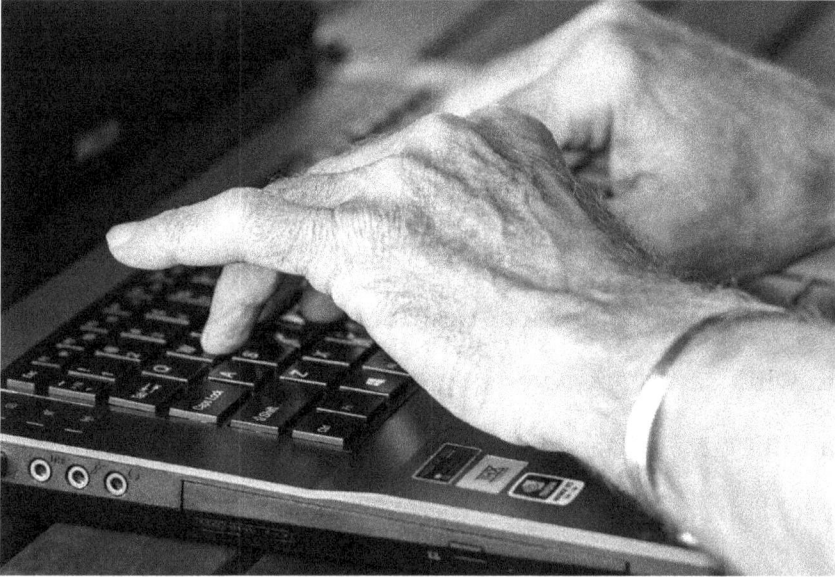

Here are some fast facts about psoriatic arthritis: Psoriatic arthritis is a persistent, progressive disease that is typified by psoriasis or an inflammation of the skin and arthritis of the joints. About 15 to 20% of patients who have psoriasis can develop this inflammation of the joints. Psoriatic arthritis can lead to spondyloarthropathies or inflammation of the spine as well as inflammation of the eyes, lung lining, cartilage and tendons. It may take years for psoriatic arthritis to first appear for patients with psoriasis characterized by low back pain, swollen joints, morning stiffness, foot pain, joint pain, swelling of fingers and toes, and reduced range of motion. Some patients suffer symptoms of conjunctivitis, nail pitting and fatigue.

Treatment of psoriatic arthritis is done autonomously of psoriasis. The usual treatments include medication, ice applications, exercise and surgery. Moreover, once people are diagnosed with psoriatic arthritis, they have a tendency to withdraw themselves from society—they suffer alone. In addition to the debilitating physical symptoms of skin problems and joint issues, the feeling of loneliness takes over their life and can affect their level of energy, their outlook in life, and their personal relationships. More than getting educated about the disease and obtaining the appropriate treatment measures, it is also important to get moral support, advice and ideas from family members, professionals and people who have been there.

Chapter One: Deeper Look at Psoriatic Arthritis

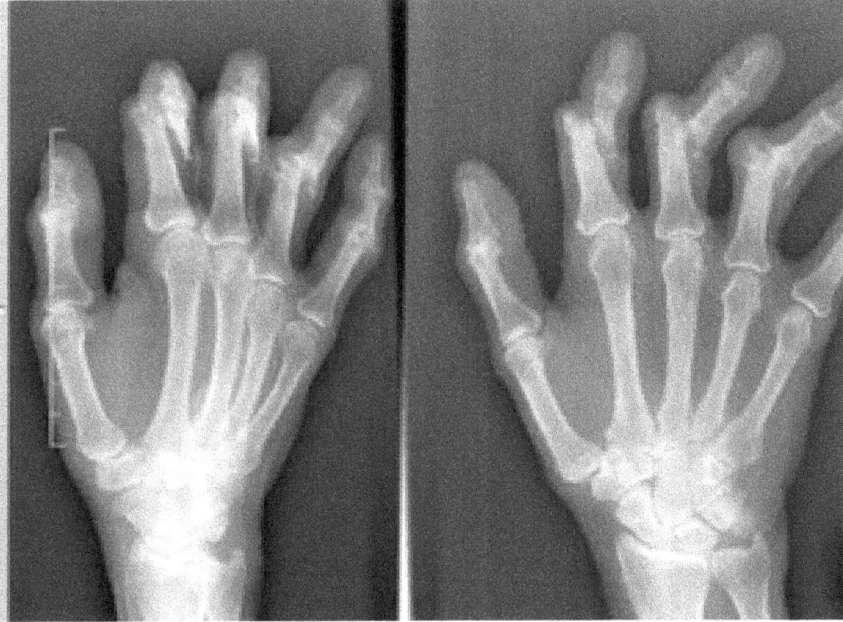

Having psoriatic arthritis is a very difficult condition. Not only do you have to deal with the symptoms of psoriasis, but you also suffer from the almost unbearable effects of arthritis. All the stiffness, swelling and discomfort in the joints can not only disrupt your daily life, but also bring tremendous amount of pain. Psoriatic arthritis is a progressive autoimmune disease. What is an autoimmune disease?

The human body has an immune system that is designed to protect itself from the onslaught of infection and disease. However, there are cases when the cells in the immune system attack healthy cells in other parts of the body by mistake—this is called autoimmune disease. There is no known cause for psoriatic arthritis just as it is not clear why autoimmune diseases develop. It is unknown as of yet why the immune system will fight healthy tissues. But the condition is likely to run in families, particularly women.

Environmental factors and physical trauma also play a vital role in the condition. The disorder in one's immune system can bring about a lower or higher rate of activity wherein tissues are damaged and the body's natural ability to ward off diseases suffer, thereby causing the body to be vulnerable to illnesses and infections. There are about 80 different kinds of autoimmune diseases and a classic symptom is inflammation. Inflammation of different kinds of body tissues can cause pain, swelling, heat, and redness, which can result in muscle aches, low fever or fatigue.

Autoimmune diseases also flare up, meaning the condition gets worse and the patient suffers remissions. The main goal of addressing autoimmune diseases is to lessen the inflammation.

As with any autoimmune disease, the symptoms of psoriatic arthritis can appear or disappear anytime. You may think that you are getting better only to suffer another, more sever flare-up of the skin and joints. Psoriasis can affect the scalp, navel, ears, knees, elbows, and even the genital areas. This inflammation of the skin is prevalent, affecting about 2% of the population of Caucasians in America. Similarly, about a quarter of patients who suffer from psoriasis can develop inflammatory arthritis.

According to studies, psoriatic arthritis begins to show in the 40s or 50s, and both males and females can be affected. The problem of skin inflammation and joint inflammation can appear separately, and usually psoriasis is the first diseases that almost 80% of people have to deal with first. In cases where the inflammatory arthritis appears first, doctors find it difficult to diagnose correctly until they develop psoriasis. In cases like this, the joint problems begin even before lesions in the skin appear.

Patients who suffer from psoriatic arthritis suffer similar symptoms of different systemic rheumatic diseases and arthritic conditions such as Crohn's disease, reactive arthritis and ankylosing spondylitis where there is inflammation of the joints, spine and some organs of the body like the heart, kidney, lungs and eyes.

Risk Factors

As with any autoimmune disease, the cause for psoriatic arthritis remains unclear. Genetics, environmental factors, family history and even physical trauma can contribute to the development of the condition. For instance, a bacterial infection can trigger the disease in people that have an inherent tendency. Following are the risk factors that can increase the possibility of developing psoriatic arthritis:

- Psoriasis. People who already have inflammation of the skin have a great chance of developing psoriatic arthritis, especially when they begin to have lesions on their nails.

- Genetics and family history. According to research, people who have relatives in the first degree that have psoriatic arthritis have a tendency to develop the illness as well.

- Age. Psoriatic arthritis tends to occur more prominently in people aged 40 to 50. Nevertheless, the condition does not only occur in this age group, anyone can acquire psoriatic arthritis.

People with psoriatic arthritis can suffer from complications. One of the most severe complications is called *arthritis mutilans*. This is a harsh, agonizing, immobilizing form of psoriatic arthritis. Arthritis mutilans will destroy the little bones like the fingers. The patient will then be disabled and deformed.

Another complication is the pinkeye or conjunctivitis. This can cause reddened eyes, blurred vision, and pain in the eye area. Depending on their genera health and the progression of the disease, some patients with psoriatic arthritis can even develop cardiovascular diseases.

Importance of Early Diagnosis

You can learn more about the different signs and symptoms of psoriatic arthritis in the next chapter. If you already have psoriasis and you start to experience joint pain, be sure to inform you doctor immediately. Early diagnosis and treatment can help you manage the condition. If untreated, the condition can relentlessly damage your joints. It is never too early to get proper treatment; it can save your life.

Rheumatologists are the ones that generally treat autoimmune diseases and psoriatic arthritis. Similarly, dermatologists, internists, general practitioners, primary care doctors and orthopedic surgeons can also be involved, depending on the patient's case. Often, occupational and physical therapists are also called upon for management.

During an examination, the doctor will closely examine your joints. He has to check if there are signs of tenderness or swelling in any of your joints. Patients usually show signs of pitting in their fingernails. There can also be flaking or other abnormalities, which can be early signs of psoriatic arthritis. The doctor will also test your soles and heels. By pressing around the areas to see if there is tenderness, he can identify if the onset of joint inflammation is underway. There is, however, no single test that can accurately diagnose the condition. The doctor will perform various tests that will help rule out other conditions that cause joint pain, for instance gout or rheumatoid arthritis. Some of the tests include x-rays, MRIs, and laboratory exams.

X-rays will help the doctor determine if there are significant changes in the joints that are only present in psoriatic arthritis and not in other arthritic disorders. An MRI (magnetic resonance imaging) will show a doctor the condition of the hard and soft tissues in the body such as ligaments and tendons in the lower back and feet. Other laboratory tests that can help identify or rule out the condition are the joint fluid tests and the rheumatoid factor.

In a joint fluid test, a sample of the joint fluid will be taken using a needle. When there is uric acid crystals in the fluid, then psoriatic arthritis may be ruled out as the condition can be gout. On the other hand, rheumatoid factor is a blood test to detect the antibody that is present in rheumatoid arthritis but is not found in psoriatic arthritis. These laboratory tests are helpful to doctors so they can properly diagnose and give appropriate treatment.

Generally speaking, there is no definite cure for psoriatic arthritis. Treatment is focused on the management of the inflammation so that the patient can control the flare-ups and prevent more pain and future disability. Usually, medications such as nonsteroidal anti-inflammatory drugs (NSAIDs), disease-modifying antirheumatic drugs (DMARDs), TNF-alpha inhibitors, immunosuppresants, and steroids are used. More treatment and management pans are discussed on another chapter of this book in detail.

Types of Psoriatic Arthritis

There are various types of psoriatic arthritis. The condition depends on the division of the joints that are disturbed by arthritis. It is important to identify the type of psoriatic arthritis that you are suffering so that the appropriate treatment regimen can be applied.

- *Spondylitis* is an inflammation of the spine. Patients that suffer from spondylitis have reduced range in motion in the neck and lower back area and they experience mild to severe pain in said areas.

- *Oligoarticular Psoriatic Arthritis* is a mild case of PsA that affects four or less of the joints in the body.

- *Polyarticular Psoriatic Arthritis* is more sever compared to oligoarticular PsA, but it also affects at least 4 joints.

- *Enthesitis* is psoriatic arthritis wherein there is swelling in the area of the tendons or ligaments. This usually happens in the spine, ribs, pelvis, and at the bottoms of the patient's feet.

- *Dactylitis* is a case of psoriatic arthritis where the fingers and toes are swollen. The fingers and toes will enlarge and the condition can cause deformities and disabilities.

- *Symmetric Psoriatic Arthritis* affects similar joints on both sides of the patient's body. For instance, both right and left knees are affected.

- *Asymmetric Psoriatic Arthritis* on the other hand, mildly affects the joints on one side of the patient's body.

- *Distal Interphalangeal Predominant Psoriatic Arthritis* is a type of Psoriatic Arthritis that affects the joints near the nails or the distal joints.

- *Psoriatic arthritis multilans* is a severe case of psoriatic arthritis that causes lower back and neck pain and affects the joints in the feet and hands.

The Future of Patients with Psoriatic Arthritis

The prognosis for psoriatic arthritis is good. Studies show that when aggressive treatment is adapted, a patient suffering from psoriatic arthritis has a good chance of improving the condition. Early diagnosis and early treatment is best, not only to avoid complications but also to give the patient a good quality of life. Conversely, if diagnosis and treatment is late, skin and joint issues can occur. Depending on the location, concentration and length of the inflammation, the patient can suffer different degrees of injury. Tissues can be destroyed and joints can become deformed. Other complications with bodily organs can also occur.

There is no known approach that can help prevent psoriatic arthritis. Treatments and pain management can help control psoriatic arthritis and stop recurrence in the future. Psoriatic is a serious condition, but the future looks bright. Treatment is evolving on a daily basis and more effective and safer medications are being formulated. Moreover, natural treatments such as lifestyle changes and diet modifications have been proven to contribute to a patient's well-being.

In summary, here are the key points: patients with psoriatic arthritis suffer from both inflammation of the skin and inflammation of the joints, so they experience stiffness, swelling, pain and reduced range of motion. The symptoms differ from person to person, some more severe than other. The most common of the symptoms include swollen and painful joints, changes in the nails, and fatigue. Two major risk factors that cause psoriatic arthritis are genetics and the environment such as viral or bacterial infections and stress. Early diagnosis and immediate treatment is necessary so that permanent damage to the patient's joints as well as complications like cardiovascular diseases and deformity can be avoided. There are conventional and natural treatments that help patients manage psoriatic arthritis.

Everyone's outlook towards psoriatic arthritis is different. Some people have mild symptoms, others have debilitating ones. The symptoms will affect your ability to move around and conduct your daily activities. It can affect not only your daily living but also your relationships and how you view life in general. Additionally, if you are diagnosed with psoriatic arthritis while you are young, it can be pretty depressing and debilitating.

Patients whose skin is covered in lesions and rashes and already have severe symptoms of psoriatic arthritis will also find it difficult to have a great outlook for the future. Nevertheless, whether you had an early or late diagnosis, or if your condition is mild or severe, it is important to obtain a good treatment regimen so that you can take back your life. Throughout this book, you will learn more about psoriatic arthritis and how you can treat it naturally or with medication, as well as get inspiration from people who have suffered the same condition. It is not too late for you to enjoy life.

Chapter Two: Signs, Symptoms and Complications

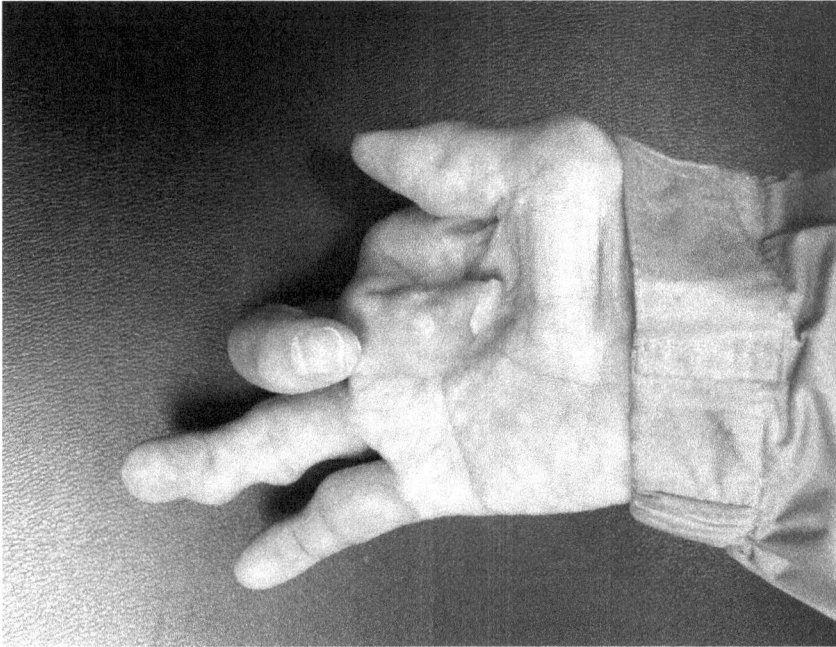

Just because you have psoriasis, doesn't mean you will develop psoriatic arthritis, regardless of the severity of your psoriasis. But the possibility is there. In that case, you should be aware of the different signs and symptoms that come with psoriatic arthritis so you can detect them and get treatment before they become worse.

Psoriatic arthritis can affect any joint in your body, and the symptom can be mild or severe. Do not think for a moment that just because the swelling or pain is slight, that the condition cannot worsen. It is best to see a doctor at the first signs of stiffness or inflammation. Here are the most common areas of inflammation that you should be on the lookout for:

Lower back pain. Pain the lower back seems to be a common problem for many people because of posture, a sedentary lifestyle, bone problems, muscle problems and the like. But it can also be caused by psoriatic arthritis, especially if you already have psoriasis. The inflammation is called spondylitis and it can affect the joints in your spine and pelvis. This can bring about pain, stiffness, weakness in the hip area, and reduced range of motion.

Foot pain. When there is pain at the soles of your feet or at the back of your heels, you may either be suffering from gout or an inflammation of your ligaments and tendons caused by psoriatic arthritis. Just to be sure, have a doctor check it out so you can get necessary treatment.

Swollen toes and fingers. Do you have a hard time moving your fingers and toes? Do you notice that your fingers and toes seem to be swelling like sausages? Go to a doctor immediately as this swelling can cause deformity if left untreated.

Swollen, tender and irritated joints. Do you feel some tenderness in your knees, elbows, shoulders, wrists, ankles? The inflammation can happen in one side or both sides of your body.

General malaise. People with psoriatic arthritis suffer from joint inflammation and oftentimes muscle tissue issues so they experience weakness, fatigue and exhaustion. The tiredness is caused by the inflammation in the body.

Reduced range of motion. The patient with psoriatic arthritis will suffer from stiff and swollen joints, thereby causing him to have reduced movements to avoid pain. You will usually experience this after doing some physical activity or when you are inactive for quite some time and start to move.

Other symptoms include morning stiffness, painful muscles, redness of the eyes, pain in your eyes, and nail pitting. Changes in the nail are more noticeable as you will see them start to separate from the nail beds, become brittle or easily break. Some symptoms are associated with psoriasis including flaky scalps and scaly skin patches, rashes and lesions. Again, it is to be noted that the symptoms and the degree of injury that come with psoriatic arthritis differ from person to person.

Left untreated, the symptoms can worsen as time goes by. Patients can suffer severe cases of anemia, deformities and disfigurements. Psoriatic arthritis is not to be overlooked as a simple condition as it can bring disability. It is a progressive disease and can lead to many complications that can not only be debilitating, but also life-threatening. Take the following into consideration:

- Joint damage, developed over time with psoriatic arthritis, is irreversible.

- Cardiovascular diseases can develop when the body is in an inflammatory state. Congestive heart failure, vascular disease, and coronary artery disease are some conditions that can develop because of inflammation. These can result in a stroke or a heart attack.

- Because of the inflammation caused by psoriatic arthritis, the auditory nerve or the inner ear can be damaged. This can bring about balance problems or hearing loss.

- Eye problems associated with inflammation include keratitis, scleritis, conjunctivitis, episcleritis, blepharitis and uveitis.

- Arthritis mutilans, as mentioned earlier, is the most severe complication patients with psoriatic arthritis have a great risk of developing. The bones in the fingers and toes can shorten, degrade, get destroyed. Not only will the patient lose function, he can also be deformed.

- There is no single medical indicator that can identify if a patient becomes susceptible to irreversible joint damage. Research suggests that the protein *calgranulin* which is found in the white blood cells, markers of angiogenesis, and certain molecules that regulate the turnover of bones can affect the condition.

Impact on One's Life

Having psoriatic arthritis can have a great impact on one's quality of life.

- The patient can suffer from physical limitations.
- School or work will be affected.
- Loss of productivity will result because of absenteeism and being unable to function properly.
- The patient will suffer from chronic fatigue.
- Psoriatic arthritis will also take a toll on one's relationships and behavior.
- The number of health care visits, hospitalizations and schedules for therapy increase as time goes by.

- Some patients may require assistive care.

- Too much suffering and pain can bring about bouts of depression.

Psoriatic arthritis is not a simple disease and it certainly does not have minimal implications on one's physical, social and mental health. That is why the importance of getting prompt treatment cannot be understated. In the following chapters, you will learn about medical treatments that can be prescribed by doctors as well as natural ways you can manage the condition. Whether it is for yourself or a loved one, do not be afraid to step out and get help.

There may be a stigma for people dealing with psoriasis or psoriatic arthritis but do not allow this stigma to hold you back from getting the right treatment you deserve. You don't have to suffer or be humiliated. Having this condition is not your fault. It is autoimmune disease—you did not do anything wrong to develop illness. But since it is already there, you have the power to overcome and manage it so you can take your life back and live fully.

If you feel any of the symptoms mentioned in this chapter, don't delay getting a check-up. Before you go to your appointment, you may want to prepare the answers to the following questions that your doctor will ask.

- What are the symptoms you are experiencing?
- When did your symptoms begin?
- What joints are affected or in pain?
- Is anyone in your immediate family affected or had a history of psoriasis or psoriatic arthritis?
- Are you taking any medications or supplements?
- Have you tried any treatment plans?
- Have the medications or treatment plans worked?
- What activities or bodily positions worsen your symptoms?

It is best to list them down so you don't forget anything. If you can go with a friend or a family member, it is also a great idea as you may not be able to remember everything that the doctor will tell you.

Chapter Three: Treatment and Management

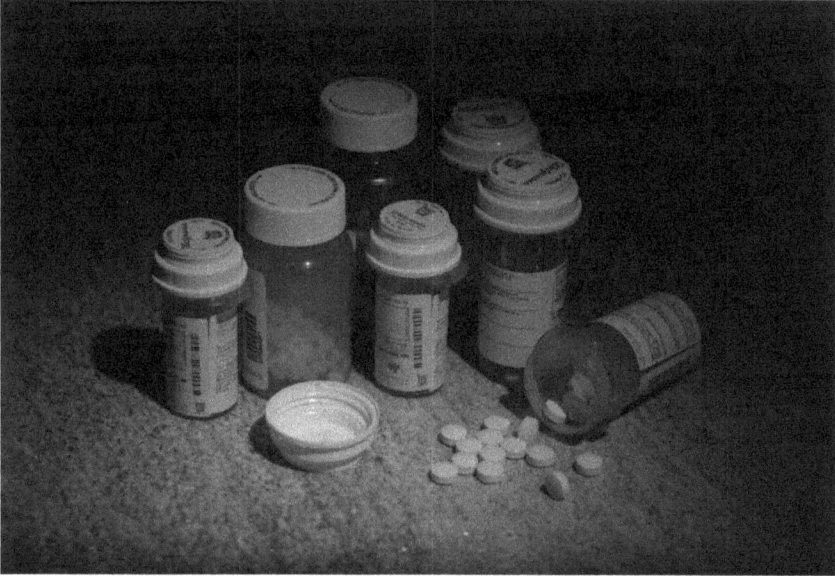

Repeatedly it is said that there is no cure for psoriatic arthritis. However, you don't have to live with its debilitating effects for the rest of your life. There are conventional treatments in place that can help you relieve the pain, reduce the swelling, lessen the stiffness and control the inflammation. The most common treatment plan that doctors advise their patients is medication. Different kinds of medication, whether prescription drugs or over-the-counter medicines, can help you manage and treat the immune response of the body that brings about inflammation. These include:

Nonsteroidal Anti-Inflammatory Drugs (NSAIDs)

NSAIDs function to diminish inflammation, pain and swelling. Some kinds of NSAI-Ds are naproxen sodium and ibuprofen; these can be bought over-the-counter. If you need stronger NSAIs, you will need prescription. While these medications can help relieve the pain and swelling, you may experience various side effects including allergic reactions, heart problems, renal damage, liver damage, and gastrointestinal -irritation. Even if you can buy it yourself, it is important to consult with a doctor first.

Immunosuppresants

To help alleviate the swelling and inflammation, doctors can prescribe arava, azathioprine, cyclosporine and methotrexate. These are immunosuppresants that inhibit the overactive immune response in your immune system that triggers the symptoms of psoriatic arthritis. However, these medications also have side effects: upset stomach, mouth sores, nausea, hair loss and liver damage. It can also increase your risk to infections because its goal is to tame your immune system.

Disease - Modifying Antirheumatic Drugs (DMARDs).

Patients with psoriatic arthritis that already suffer from progressive joint damage are given the more aggressive medication DMARDs. This is done to prevent deformity and eventual joint destruction. However, the use of DMARDs can result in the risk of suppression of the bone marrow and liver damage. When a patient is administered with DMARDs, their blood count should be regularly monitored and liver blood tests should be undertaken.

Corticosteroids

These medications help reduce the inflammation in the joints as well as the pain and swelling. Corticosteroids suppress the inflammatory pathways in your body, mimicking the body's hormone cortisol, produced by the adrenal glands. You can take corticosteroids by mouth or by local injections. The most common corticosteroids are methylprednisolone, dexamethasone, and prednisone. It provides immediate but temporary relief from the pain. With long term use, the side effects associated with corticosteroids include infections, easy bruising, thinning of the skin, diabetes, weight gain, face swelling, osteoporosis, weak bones or even bone death.

TNF inhibitors

These are anti-tumor necrosis factor agents that doctors prescribe to patients who suffer from both psoriasis and psoriatic arthritis. TNF inhibitors s can ease the pain and swelling, relieve the stiffness and even improve the tissues of the skin. This medication is usally prescribed for those who have severe cases of psoriatic arthritis. The most common TNF inhibitors include infliximab (Remicade), etanercept (Enbrel), golimumab (Simponi), certolizumab pegol (Cimzia) and adalimumab (Humira). TNF inhibitors can suppress psoriasis and arthritis and even prevent progressive joint injury. The risk for infection is increased, however, with the intake of such medications whether they are given through injections or intravenously. Other side effects include skin reactions, low blood pressure and breathing problems.

Therapy and Surgery as Conventional Treatment

Along with medication, physical and occupational therapy is prescribed for patients with psoriatic arthritis to prevent the degeneration of joints as well as to bring mobility and reduce pain. Exercises are critical components of treatment plans for psoriatic arthritis. With physical activity, a patient's joint movement will be maintained and disability will be prevented.

Low-impact exercises can be beneficial in improving the patients' well-being and mobility. When the patient is exposed to physical activity, muscle strength is improved as well, so that doing daily tasks becomes easy. Following are the exercises that can help with a patient's range of motion:

-   Stretching. Exercises such as Yoga and Tai Chi involve a lot of stretching that can improve flexibility of muscles and increase the range of motion in a person's joints. By doing stretching exercises regularly, even the simplest ones, a person with psoriatic arthritis can prevent stiffness and keep himself mobile.

-   Strength Training. It is important to strengthen bones and muscles so that you can prevent osteoporosis and develop more stable joints. Therapists can require use of resistance bands and dumbbells. Lifting weights and doing Pilates exercises will also help strengthen a patient's body.

-   Aerobic Exercises. A patient suffering from psoriatic arthritis needs to enhance his physical endurance. Walking, jogging, cycling and swimming will not only increase endurance and stamina but also improve a person's mood, decrease inflammation and bring about more energy. Doing aerobic exercises also bring cardiovascular benefits.

The symptoms of psoriatic arthritis can diminish or flare up at any moment. By moving and stretching, the pain, swelling, stiffness and inflammation can lessen.

Another kind therapeutic treatment is light therapy. Psoriatic arthritis patients are exposed to natural UV ultraviolet light and artificial UV ultraviolet light. According to research, the combination of both UV lights not only treats the skin, but also makes the joints respond positively. The use of light therapy is suggested for patients with mild cases of skin and joint issues.

The relationship of psoriasis and psoriatic arthritis is still unclear, but studies have shown that the arthritis manifestations clear up when the skin inflammation is addressed. Similarly, exposure to direct sunlight, vitamin D, can also benefit patients with psoriasis and psoriatic arthritis.

In severe cases of psoriatic arthritis, where joints have suffered acute damage, surgery may be required. Patients may need to have knee joint replacements, hip joint replacements, or other orthopedic surgical repairs. Artificial prostheses can replace severely damaged joints.

The seriousness of psoriatic arthritis cannot be undermined. However, clinical trials and medical advancements happen on a daily basis. These help doctors and medical professionals get a better understanding of how the body responds to autoimmune diseases such as psoriatic arthritis. More, newer therapies are being developed and treatment plans are being made to control the inflammation, mitigate discomfort, and slow down or totally stop the progression of psoriatic arthritis symptoms.

If you are not inclined to pharmacological treatments, you can go about treating symptoms of psoriatic arthritis through natural means. Or you may want to employ alternative remedies to complement pharmacological means. Read on to the next chapter to discover different means on how you can effectively reduce the inflammation, treat symptoms and manage psoriatic arthritis without medication and the fear of side effects.

Chapter Four: Dealing with Psoriatic Arthritis Naturally

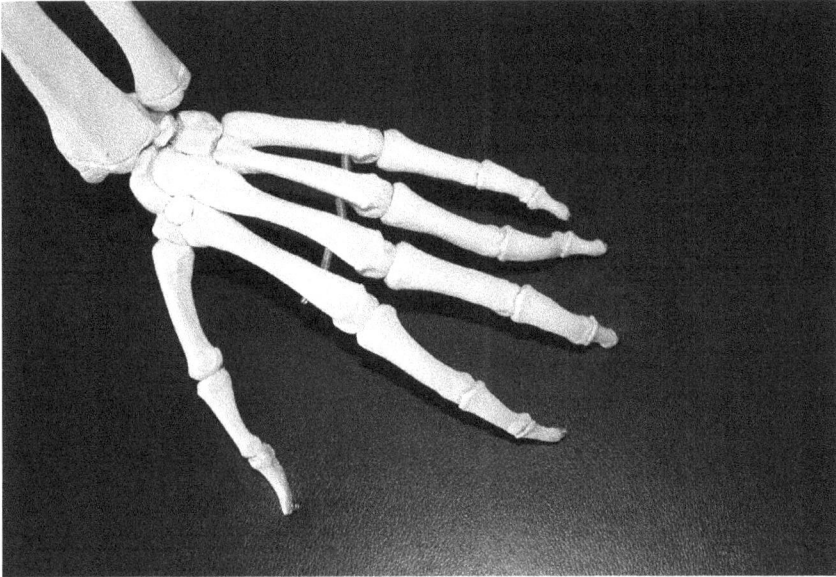

The progress of psoriatic arthritis can be stalled by medication and traditional therapies, causing the symptoms to ease up. However, there are also alternative, natural means that you can apply to complement these treatment plans. Many people feel more in control of their life and their condition when they can do something naturally to improve psoriatic arthritis symptoms.

This chapter will discuss various lifestyle and home remedies that you can implement in your daily life. Some of them may sound too simple, but they are nonetheless effective. Most of them will be lifestyle changes that will help you protect your joints. These are the most affected by psoriatic arthritis that is why changing the way you do things everyday like lifting, pushing, and the likes, will bring about a great positive impact to your physical and mental condition.

Avoid inflammatory food

This is very basic. There are different kinds of foods that trigger inflammation of tissues and you should do your best to avoid them. Alcohol, sugar, trans - fat and caffeine are the most common triggers of inflammation. For other people, taking in dairy, gluten and shellfish can cause a reaction or sensitivity that can lead to inflammation. By eating a balanced diet and staying away from inflammatory foods, you will reduce the risk of swelling and stiffness significantly. You should also eat more anti-inflammatory foods such as broccoli, green leafy vegetables, pineapple, blueberries and walnuts. Instead of trans - fat, go for healthy fats like coconut oil and avocado. Eat good quality protein such as organic chicken, grass-fed beef and salmon caught from the wild. Quinoa, brown rice and oats are also a healthy option. If you think about it, your diet won't be too limited at all. And if you consider the good effects on your body—you don't have to worry about pain and inflammation—then you will have all the motivation you need to avoid inflammatory foods.

Lose the extra pounds

Additional weight puts in a stress in your joints. When you are too heavy, it is easy for your joints to get inflamed. People who are obese, overweight or have metabolic syndromes often suffer from psoriatic arthritis. If they are given DMARDs to address the Psoriatic Arthritis, the medication may not be as effective.

When you maintain a healthy weight, there is less chance for swelling and stiffness. Not only that, you will also improve your flexibility, mobility and energy. Get into the habit of having a healthy, anti-inflammatory and balanced diet and a good exercise regimen to maintain a good weight. Eat a good amount of vegetables, fruits, and whole grains so you can limit your calories while increasing the nutrient intake of your body. Maintaining your weight has greater health benefits other than easing symptoms of psoriatic arthritis. Don't forget, health is wealth.

Be active.

Living a sedentary lifestyle has many downsides. It is bad not only for people with psoriatic arthritis but for all kinds of people. Everyone needs to move and exercise to stay healthy, maintain a good range of motion, avoid stiffness, prevent inflammation and improve their flexibility. Even the simplest of exercises such as jogging and walking can give so many benefits. Try biking, swimming, and aerobics. You don't have to go to the gym all the time. What's important is to keep your body moving. It can alleviate the pain that comes with symptoms of psoriatic arthritis. Not only will you improve your physical condition, you will also boost your mental health. Exercise is known to improve moods and boost energy. If you don't have the will to exercise on your own, get a partner or a therapist to work with you. This way you can improve your performance and you also get the benefit of emotional support and motivation. Besides, there is no health benefit to being a couch potato.

Avoid stress

Studies show that stress can cause inflammation. In today's world where everything is fast-paced and stressful, you need to know how to manage stress levels and triggers. Many researches show that stress is a contributing factor to different autoimmune diseases. Stress can trigger inflammatory cellular reactions in the body and causes an imbalance. That is the best reason why you should learn to reduce stress in your life.

First, you need to know what triggers your stress reactions. Is it work, your environment, the people you interact with? What things can you eliminate in your life in order to reduce stress? If you cannot remove these triggers from your life, you need to know how you can control yourself and manage these conditions so that they do not affect you adversely. Some ways you can manage stress are yoga, meditation, taking nature walks, prayer, writing journals, listening to music or going on vacations. You can also do aromatherapy, get a massage or use essential oils. However you choose to do it, you need to unwind and minimize the stress levels around you so that you can avoid inflammation. Stress-reducing activities should be incorporated into your daily life.

Pace yourself.

When you suffer from psoriatic arthritis, the effects of inflammation can leave you exhausted. The same is true when you are taking medication. But this doesn't mean that you should stop being active because you feel fatigue. The best way is to pace yourself—you need to rest before your body becomes too tired. Divide your work and exercise into brisk segments so that you can relax in between. Never push yourself too much or even the medications you take won't bring you relief from the pain and swelling. Pacing has never killed anyone, so don't be afraid to move slower and steadier.

Get support.

It will be hard to cope with pain and inflammation on a daily basis, especially if your symptoms are severe. The emotional and mental pain brought by psoriatic arthritis can equal or even be greater than the physical pain. Don't be afraid or embarrassed to get the support of family members and friends to help you cope. If you can find a support group near your area, you can get the same motivational benefits that will help you get through the challenges of your condition. You can also seek professional help from a counselor or therapist.

He can help you manage your stress levels. Remember, stress can aggravate the symptoms of psoriatic arthritis. You can even go for lifestyle counselling especially when you have alcohol intake or smoking issues, as well as weight loss counselling. By being able to talk with someone and have someone help you do things that can address your condition, you won't feel too burdened by psoriatic arthritis.

Being brave doesn't mean you don't ask for help. You don't have to go through it alone. There will always be someone to help you.

Acupuncture

One form of complementary therapy that you can apply is acupuncture. The method has been known to help relieve neck pain, back pain, shoulder pain, joint pain and knee pain. Acupuncture has been used for more than 5,000 years and it is a way to release the natural hormones in the body that kills pain, namely adenosine, serotonin and endorphins. That is why it is one of the best means to help psoriasis and psoriatic arthritis. It is a proven safe treatment that will not obstruct other existing treatments for psoriatic arthritis, including medications.

Epsom salts

For people that do not like medications and the side effects that come with them, natural pain killers are the best option. Epsom salts can help reduce inflammation and alleviate pain in the joints. To take an Epsom bath, add Epsom salts to warm bath water and soak in it for 15 minutes. The magnesium in Epsom salts will calm the itchiness and remove the scales in the skin. It will also bring soothing comfort to your joints.

Turmeric

Turmeric has potent anti-inflammatory properties. The curcumin in turmeric is also an antioxidant. There are many variations of turmeric that you can take: turmeric tea, dietary supplement, turmeric powder that you can add to a teaspoon of honey, or turmeric essential oil that you can add to water. Some research shows that taking about 1000 mg a day of curcumin helps relieve joint arthritis symptoms.

Massage therapy

Getting a massage can help relax your muscles. It will also help alleviate the pain in your joints and reduce the stiffness and swelling. It is also a good way to release stress. Go to a massage therapist that is professionally trained in dealing with psoriatic arthritis so that he can address the tight joints and muscles and relieve the discomfort.

Vitamin supplements

Some doctors can prescribe supplements for vitamins and minerals that can help you become healthier and develop a stronger immune system. These include vitamin D, calcium, and folic acid. Omega-3 fish oil supplements are also good for inflammatory diseases. Some patients who take regular omega-3 fatty acid supplements were said to use less painkillers.

Oats

Often the pain of psoriatic arthritis is aggravated by the pain and irritation on the skin caused by psoriasis. Soaking in an oat bath, making an oat paste or using oat soaps can help relieve the itchy patches. It can soothe the skin and bring down the heat.

Apple cider vinegar

A lot of people think apple cider vinegar is a miracle cure-all. While that may be contested, the good effects of apple cider vinegar for weight loss and for treating psoriasis cannot be devalued. Apple cider vinegar can be applied to patches of psoriasis in the scalp and this can help relieve any pain and irritation. However, apple cider vinegar should not be applied to areas of the skin that are bleeding and cracked.

Tea tree oil

Like apple cider vinegar, tea tree essential oil can also help relieve pain and irritation from skin lesions caused by psoriasis. However, you should check first because tea tree oil may not be good for sensitive skin.

Capsaicin

Capsaicin blocks pain receptors in the body. You can get over-the-counter creams that contain capsaicin and use it as a soothing balm to address pain and stiffness caused by inflammation.

Managing psoriatic arthritis may involve a combination of pharmacological and alternative means. It can also be addressed by natural means. The best choice is dependent on the severity of the psoriatic arthritis of the patient, any prior treatment or medication undertaken and other conditions. Likewise, it is largely the patient's choice that is the determining factor. It is best to keep in mind that natural remedies are not a total substitute for prescribed treatments. It is always good to consult with medical professionals first. Whatever type of pain management is undertaken, as long as the condition is addressed early and appropriately, the progression of the disease can be stalled and deformity can be prevented.

Homeopathic Treatment

Some patients prefer homeopathic treatments to deal with their psoriatic arthritis. While it is a safe alternative, and can improve the patient's quality of life, it is still best to consult with a medical professional first regarding your condition. Moreover, homeopathic treatment should be done by a homeopathic doctor after a thorough examination.

Depending on the severity of the disease and the family history, homeopathic medicines can be desirable and can bring a positive response on different tissues. If you are not using conventional medicines, homeopathy may work well for you. If you are on the early stages of psoriatic arthritis, then homeopathy can bring you quick relief. Some of the homeopathy medicines that can treat psoriatic arthritis include Radium bromatum, Rhus toxicodendron, Thuja occidentalis, Ledum palustre and Kali carbonicum. These can reduce stiffness and minimize inflammation as well as relieve a patient's pain. Homeopathic medicines can also stop the progress of psoriatic arthritis so people can improve the quality of their life. When the cause of the pain is treated, the symptoms of psoriatic arthritis will be relieved.

Chapter Five: How Changing Your Diet can Affect Psoriatic Arthritis

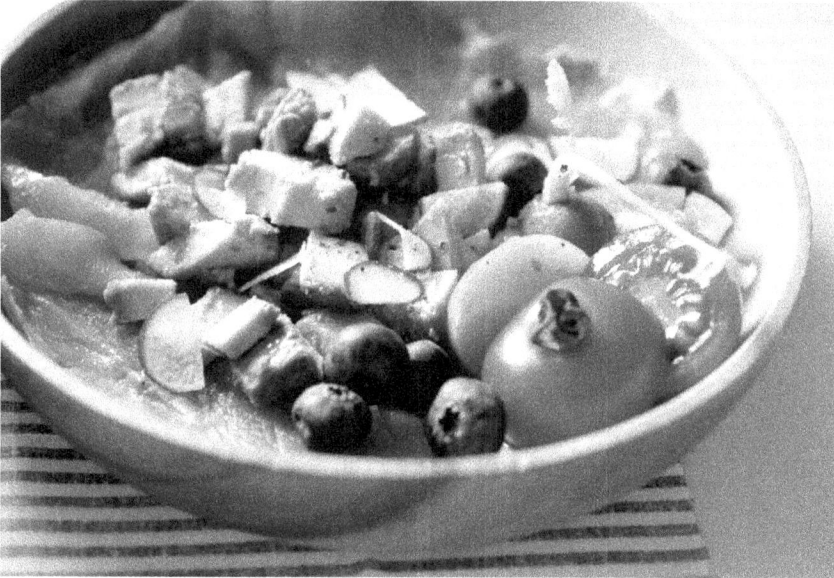

Eating healthy has always been the best way to prevent illnesses and to improve any condition. This is especially true for patients who have psoriatic arthritis. Some of the basic tips include eating a good amount of vegetables and fruits, eating good protein from lean meat, choosing whole grains, eating fat-free or low-fat products, and drinking a lot of water.

Could changing one's diet really improve the conditions of psoriatic arthritis? The answer is yes. Simply because when you avoid inflammatory foods, you easily avoid swelling and stiffness. You will experience milder symptoms. And you will have lesser physical and emotional pain that is associated with the condition. If only for that reason, then you should change your diet.

Here are some popular diets that you can adopt, along with lists of foods you need to avoid. How they can help with psoriatic arthritis is also discussed.

Anti-Inflammatory Diet

As discussed previously in lifestyle changes you need to apply, psoriatic arthritis can cause swelling. The inflammation can be triggered by the following:

- fatty foods
- fried foods
- red meat

- processed foods

- refined sugars

- dairy

- certain vegetables like potato and eggplant.

- refined carbohydrates like white bread and pastries

- French fries

- soda and other sugar-sweetened drinks

- margarine, shortening, and lard

- vegetable oil

- refined flour

- artificial sweeteners

- artificial additives

- saturated fats

If you avoid these foods, you avoid causing inflammation. Go for non-inflammatory foods instead. An anti-inflammatory diet includes the following foods to eat: foods high in antioxidants and omega-3 fatty acids such as:

- Avocados

- Apples

- Artichokes

- Berries (such as blueberries, black berries, and raspberries)
- Beans (such as black beans, red beans, and pinto beans)
- Broccoli
- Cherries
- Dark chocolate (at least 70 percent cocoa)
- Dark green leafy vegetables (such as spinach, kale, and collard greens)
- Nuts (such as almonds, walnuts, hazelnuts and pecans)
- Whole grains (such as oats, brown rice and quinoa)
- Sweet potatoes
- Omega-3-fortified foods (including eggs and milk)
- Oily fish (such as mackerel, salmon, sardines, tuna, herring, and anchovies)
- Flaxseed
- Walnuts
- Turmeric
- Ginger
- Garlic

Here is a meal idea for an anti-inflammatory diet:

- For breakfast, you can have an oatmeal bowl, a breakfast smoothie or a chia bowl.
- For lunch, you can eat grilled salmon, salad with quinoa and vegetables and soup.
- Snacks can include apples and nut butter, chia seed pudding or fresh blueberry fruit salad.
- Drinks can include golden milk, green smoothie, herbal tea, or ginger turmeric tea

If you are going to follow an anti-inflammatory diet, you should:

- Daily, eat 5 – 9 servings of vegetables and fruits that are rich in antioxidants.
- Take foods high in omega-3 and not onega-6 fatty acids.
- Avoid red meat and replace them with lean poultry, soy, fish, and beans.
- Use olive oil instead of margarine and vegetable oils.

- Use whole grains instead of refined grains. You can have oats, quinoa, pastas and brown rice.
- Instead of seasoning your food with salt, use garlic, turmeric and ginger as spices.

Paleo Diet

The Paleo diet is also known as the "caveman diet". Paleo dieters favor eating meat and fish. In the Paleo diet, you will have to avoid beans, grains, dairy and sugary snacks. When you avoid eating fatty, sugary and dairy foods, you can avoid swelling and inflammation associated with psoriatic arthritis.

This diet is based on what was supposedly eaten during the Paleolithic era, about 10,000 to 2.5 million years ago. The purpose of the diet is to return to the way early humans ate, with the belief that the body is genetically mismatched to the kinds of foods that are available now. Foods to eat include:

- Vegetables

- Fruits

- Nuts

- Seeds

- Eggs

- Lean meats, preferably wild game or grass-fed

- Fish like albacore tuna, mackerel and salmon (rich in omega-3 fatty acids)

- Oils from nuts and fruits like walnut or olive oil

Foods to avoid include

- Salt

- Potatoes

- Dairy products

- Grains like oats, barley and wheat

- Legumes like peanuts, lentils, peas and beans

- Potatoes

- Processed foods

A sample menu for a Paleo diet is:

- For breakfast, you can eat cantaloupe and broiled
  salmon
- For lunch, vegetable salad (can be romaine lettuce
  with tomatoes, cucumber and carrots and lemon juice
  dressing) and broiled lean pork
- For dinner, lean beef roast, steamed broccoli and
  strawberries
- Snacks can include carrot sticks, celery sticks or
  orange fruit

Other than helping reduce the incidents of inflammation,
a Paleo diet can also bring the following benefits: better
weight loss, better blood pressure, improved glucose
tolerance, lower triglycerides and better management of
your appetite.

Gluten - Free Diet

Studies show that about a quarter of people who
suffer from psoriasis and psoriatic arthritis are sensitive to
gluten. Gluten is a kind of protein that is found in barley and

wheat used to thicken food. There is no gluten in vegetables,

fruit, meat, and dairy. Here is a list of grains that are gluten-

free:

- Rice
- Arrowroot
- Corn (maize)
- Amaranth
- Beans
- Flax
- Cassava
- Chia
- Yucca
- Millet
- Soy
- Sorghum
- Quinoa
- Potato
- Tapioca
- Buckwheat groats (also known as kasha)
- Teff

- Gluten-free oats

- Nut flours

Some of the things you need to avoid are:

- Cereals. A lot of cereals have wheat-based ingredients
  and have gluten. Always check the label. Puffed rice
  and corn flakes, which contain malt, also has gluten.

- Oats. Oats can be contaminated with gluten as they
  are harvested with the same farming equipment used
  with wheat. Even granola bars can have gluten so
  aways check if the products are labeled as gluten-free.

- Prepared Soups and Sauces. These contain hidden
  gluten, particularly cream-based canned soups and
  sauces.

Most beverages like sodas, sports drinks and juices are
gluten-free. Wines, hard liquors, hard ciders and other
alcoholic beverages are also gluten-free. But malt beverages,
ales, beers, lagers, and malt vinegars contain gluten.

Similarly, not all vitamin supplements and medicines are gluten-free, it is best to read the label to make sure.

Mediterranean Diet

A diet that contains a high amount of extra virgin olive oil has been known to diminish the symptoms of psoriatic arthritis. Omega-3 rich foods relieve the swelling. However, before you start a Mediterranean diet, you need to have a doctor check you up first, because it can either worsen or improve your symptoms, depending on your condition.

This kind of diet plan will emphasizes eating plant-based foods, whole grains, nuts and legumes. You will also use herbs and spices to replace salt and MSG to add flavor to your food. Similarly, it requires that you get enough exercise and drink red wine moderately even as you reduce your red meat intake and replace butter with healthier oils. Basically you will:

- Eat: cold-water fish, seafood, fruits, vegetables, tubers, nuts, seeds, legumes, breads, whole grains, herbs, spices, and extra virgin olive oil.
- Eat in moderation: poultry, eggs, dairy.
- Eat only rarely: red meat.

Here is a sample list of the foods you can eat:

- Fish and seafood: Salmon, mackerel, trout, tuna, sardines, oysters, shrimp, clams, mussels, crab, etc.
- Vegetables: Brussels sprouts, tomatoes, kale, spinach, cauliflower, broccoli, onions, carrots, cucumbers, etc.
- Fruits: Apples, oranges, strawberries, pears, bananas, grapes, figs, melons, dates, peaches, etc.
- Nuts and seeds: Almonds, cashews, walnuts, hazelnuts, sunflower seeds, macadamia nuts, pumpkin seeds, etc.
- Legumes: Beans, peanuts, lentils, peas, pulses, chickpeas, etc.
- Tubers: Potatoes, turnips, sweet potatoes, yams, etc.

- Whole grains: Whole oats, corn, rye, barley, brown rice, buckwheat, whole wheat, whole-grain bread and pasta.
- Herbs and spices: Garlic, mint, cinnamon, rosemary, pepper, basil, sage, nutmeg, etc.
- Healthy Fats: Extra virgin olive oil, avocados, olives, and avocado oil.
- Poultry: Chicken, turkey, duck, etc.
- Eggs: Chicken, duck and quail eggs.
- Dairy: Cheese, yogurt, Greek yogurt, etc.

You will avoid:

- Added sugar found in candies, ice cream, soda, table sugar and the likes
- Refined grains such as pasta made with refined wheat, white bread, etc.
- Trans - fats from processed foods and margarine
- Refined oils such as canola oil, soybean oil, and cottonseed oil
- All processed meats

- All highly processed foods especially those that are
  labeled "low-fat" or "diet" foods

Weight Loss Diet

One of the most important diets you can do to
alleviate inflammation and symptoms of psoriatic arthritis is
a weight loss diet. People who are obese and overweight
have a greater risk of suffering from psoriatic arthritis. When
you maintain a good weight, you lose the fat tissues that
release the proteins that trigger inflammation.

A weight loss diet consists of healthy foods such as
fruits, vegetables, fish, legumes, nuts and seeds. Avocado
oil, extra virgin coconut oil and unrefined coconut oil is also
good for cooking healthful foods. Seasoning should be done
using fresh herbs and spices such as rosemary, cinnamon,
oregano, turmeric, garlic, ginger and sage. You should limit
your intake of sugars, carbohydrates and fats. Not only will
you lose extra, unwanted pounds, you will also minimize
the risk of cancer, diabetes and heart disease. Moreover, you

will have increased mobility and you will feel much, much

better.

Other foods that are good include matcha or green

tea, avocado, leafy greens, fatty fish and ginger. Food to

avoid include cakes and cookies, packaged snack foods

white bread, white rice, processed or enriched bread

products, sugary drinks and soda, processed meats such as

bacon, hotdogs and sausages, candy, fried foods, sugary

drinks and alcohol.

Maintaining a Healthy Gut

You are what you eat has some truth to it. If you eat

heathy, you will be healthy. Eat junk and you will

experience all sorts of illnesses. When you keep your gut

healthy, your overall health will improve. Your immune

system will stabilize and be strong, you will have good

metabolism and you will maintain a healthful weight. With

the right kinds and amounts of food, the bacteria in your gut

will stay healthy and will be able to perform its crucial role.

Some studies show that a person's diet will directly
impact the community of bacteria in the gut. People with
psoriatic arthritis have a less diverse community of good gut
bacteria and therefore have more inflammations. Low-fiber
and simple carbohydrate diets can starve the healthful
bacteria. You may have an unhealthy gut if you experience
the following symptoms:

- chronic constipation
- chronic diarrhea
- being sick multiple times a year
- prolonged symptoms of sickness
- recent use of antibiotics
- autoimmune conditions

To keep your gut healthy, make sure you get a good
variety of vegetables and fruits, fermented fruits, beans and
legumes and probiotics. Fermented foods include kefir,
kombucha, Kimchi, sauerkraut, and miso.

In conclusion, there is no single diet that is prescribed for patients with psoriatic arthritis. A good diet will be something that consists of anti-inflammatory foods that will decrease the prevalence of the symptoms of psoriatic arthritis, reduce inflammation and stop complications. Eating healthy is one step to staying healthy. Another thing you can do as a lifestyle change that you can add to healthy eating is to adjust your posture. When you do this, you will effectively minimize the strain on the joints. Don't forget to do stretches and simple exercises to improve your mobility. When you do these two simple lifestyle changes, you can bring great improvement to a life with psoriatic arthritis.

Chapter Five: How Changing Your Diet Can Affect Psoriatic Arthritis

Chapter Six: Living with Psoriatic Arthritis

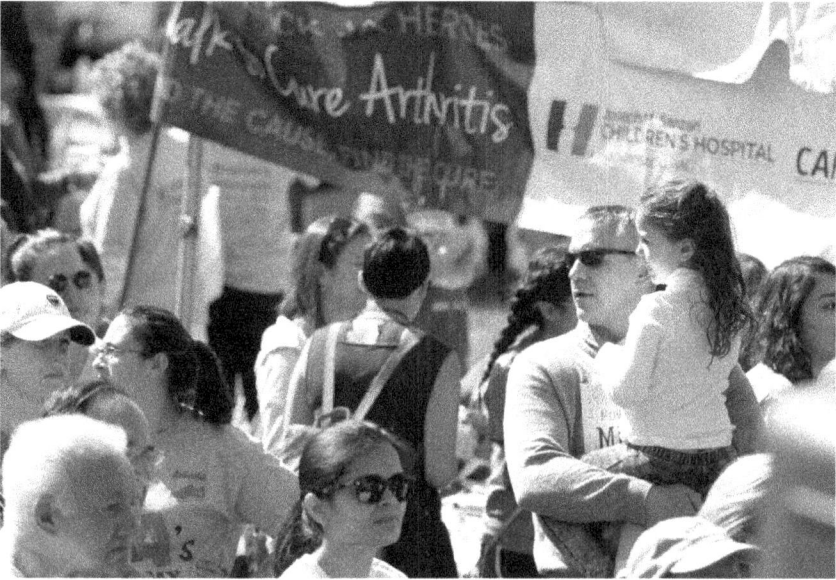

So you have psoriatic arthritis. It doesn't mean that you are a disabled person nor should you look down on yourself. If, on the other hand, you live with someone who has psoriatic arthritis, read on to find out tips on how you help them can live a better life even if they have the disease.

Tips for People with Psoriatic Arthritis

1. Learn to maintain flexibility.

   If you are going through physical or occupational therapy, make sure that you do the simple exercises that are taught you at home. The simple stretches as well as the gentle movements will be good for your joints and mobility, especially if you have been sitting or not moving for long periods of time. Don't overdo it, though.

2. Make sure you distribute loads.

   It is crucial that you don't do anything to injure your joints. If you have psoriatic arthritis, your joints are highly susceptible to damage. When you are carrying something, pushing or pulling, it is important that you protect your joints by moving properly. When you are carrying groceries, your child, or other heavy things, you should distribute the weight evenly so that there is no too much pressure on just one joint. Always use two hands when you carry something and do not just carry your bag on one shoulder. These simple things can go a long way in helping you keep your joints safe.

3. Use hot and cold therapy.

   Use cold therapy or ice therapy when your joints are hot. When your joints are stiff, use warm compress. Always remember to cover the ice packs with a towel so that you won't burn your skin. An electric heating pad is a good heat therapy method and is safer than hot water bottles. You can also use a gel-filled heat pack or a heat lamp. You can get a good soak in a warm bath to soothe the joints. You can also get massages to relieve the stiffness and aching joints.

4. Reduce your stress.

   One of the lifestyle changes to manage your stress. As discussed in detail previously, stress is never good for anyone. Make sure you do stress management techniques daily. Other things to do to help you reduce stress include: avoiding caffeine, alcohol, and nicotine, indulging in physical activity, getting more sleep, talking to someone about your condition, taking control of your life and schedule by managing your time, and keeping a stress diary.

5. Respect your limitations.

    Never push yourself. You need to learn to listen to your joints. Even if you want to do something so bad, when you feel that your joints are suffering, just stop. Nothing is more important than keeping your joints safe and mobile. When you lose it, it's gone and you can't get them back. Similarly, when you don't move them, you also face the risk of damage. How do you know when you should move and when you should rest? When your joints feel achy and they are stiff, that it's the time to gently move and mobilize them. When you feel that they are swollen and tender, then you should rest them as much as you can. Exercise can relieve the symptoms of psoriatic arthritis, but you have to consider how your joints are feeling at the moment, especially when they are tired and in pain. You can't just jump to exercising. You have to understand where your body is at present before you build it up.

6. Take pain medications as needed and prescribed. Even if you believe in the power of natural remedies, don't be afraid to take pain medication when absolutely necessary. Not all medications are bad for the body, even if there are some side effects. Some of them can reduce pain significantly and allow you to go about your day with ease. Talk to a doctor and get the best pain medication you can find.

   Remember to always bring your medication with you as you don't know when the psoriatic arthritis symptoms will flare up. Always have them on hand so that you can get them or someone can get them for you easily. Don't go out of the house without your prescribed medications. It will make your life easier.

7. Wear good shoes.

    Patients with psoriatic arthritis suffer from foot
    problems as well as pain in their ankles. Often, your
    ankles will be swollen and you won't be able to fit
    them in regular shoes. Make sure that you get and
    wear good shoes so that you don't have to suffer the
    pain in your feet. There are shoes that have a high toe
    box. You can also use shoe inserts and heel cups. Or
    you can get a shoe size that is wider than your normal
    size. These simple things will help in your daily
    activities as you will relieve foot pain. If, however,
    changing shoe sizes and using inserts or soft pads
    won't work for you, it is best to visit a podiatrist for a
    more specific solution.

8. Take daily power naps.

    Never underestimate the power of a short rest. They
    are not called power naps for no reason. You need
    that extra burst of energy especially when you are
    dealing with pain and inflammation the whole day.
    The symptoms of psoriatic arthritis can cause fatigue

even to the strongest and healthiest of people. To make sure that you don't suffer from chronic fatigue and weakness, take short breaks and get some power naps. A ten or fifteen-minute nap can do wonders not just to your body, but to your mind and emotions as well.

Getting extra rest is very important especially for people with a heavy workload, busy schedules or those with kids. But you can't just stop everything — that is why you need to pace yourself. Don't do too many things at one don't take on more than you can handle, take good amounts of rest during the day and get enough sleep. Think about it, the chores can wait. If you get overcome by fatigue, you won't be able to function well anyway. If you need to take a sick day, take it. Your health is more important than any to-do list.

9. Focus on positive things.

Positivity has often helped improved many health conditions, whether physical or mental. The same is true for cases of psoriatic arthritis. It won't be an easy journey and it will be highly likely that you may often feel lonely and tired. You can draw inspiration from your family, especially if you have children. You can practice mindfulness meditation. Always look for the silver lining. Find someone who can speak life and motivation into you. You don't have to give up. There are still so many good things about life that you can enjoy and when you focus on the positive things, you will bring a lightness into your life and reduce any form of stress that can trigger inflammation or other symptoms.

10. Ask for help (or be the help).

A lot of people who suffer from psoriatic arthritis would rather just call in sick instead of ask for help when they feel that the symptoms are affecting their ability to work. Talk with your superior about making necessary adjustments that can help you function better while at work. If you are someone who works with or lives with a person suffering from psoriatic arthritis, ask them what kind of help they need so that they can function better and with ease. Offer as much help as you can. For instance, don't place everyday items into high shelves or cabinets; make sure that tables and chairs are ergonomic, etc. These may be little things, but they can ring great relief to people with swollen or stiff joints and reduced range of mobility. The less these people struggle with pain, the less the possibility of flare ups.

You think these tips are easy? Yes, they are. But they can bring remarkable increase to the quality of your daily life as you deal with psoriatic arthritis. But here is the most important thing: nothing will happen and you will get no benefit simply by reading. You need to get started today! Life with psoriatic arthritis can be difficult, but it can be managed. Some days can be tougher than others, but stay strong and keep on going. It is also advisable to check in regularly with your doctor or therapist so that your progress can be monitored and other problems can be avoided. Sometimes, all you need is just a little tweak in your medication or physical therapy and your symptoms can be reduced significantly.

Travel Tips for People with Psoriatic Arthritis

Everyday living can already be difficult for people with psoriatic arthritis. And it can even be more difficult when they travel. But this doesn't mean they will just have to stay where they are and not enjoy going around. All you need to do is take extra careful measures. Here are some tips that you can use in planning, packing and travelling to make your future trips a success:

Don't forget to pack everything you may need. Of course, top priority on your packing list is your pain medication. It is difficult to travel, especially if you are going on long distances, if you have psoriatic arthritis. The discomfort can trigger a flare up, especially if you will sit for long periods whether by plane or car. The joint can become stiff or swollen in this condition, making the travel unbearable and also can lead to mental stress. That is why it is important to have your medication handy. Also have your doctor's contact information ready should you need to contact the office and pharmacy.

Make sure that before your trip, you have enough medication with you. If you have injectable medication, or those that need to be refrigerated, airport security may require a letter from your doctor. Pack some hand cream that can soothe dry skin as well as some essential oils that can help you relax. Make sure you have water to keep you hydrated. If you can also pack a heat pack or a cold gel, you can use it for when a flare up happens. Bring a travel pillow so that you won't suffer from neck or back pains. It is also a good idea to bring your favorite tunes along with you as they can help you relax during the trip. Make sure you pack everything you need to help you manage your condition.

More importantly, use lightweight luggage that has wheels. This will make carrying your things easier for you. Don't bring too many heavy things. Pack comfortable, loose-fitting clothes which will make you feel good and light.

Should you need special accommodations, don't hesitate to advise your carrier or travel company. This way, you can get assistance with carrying your luggage, get a more comfortable aisle seat and even arrange for a wheelchair ahead of time.

When travelling in different modes of transportation:

o By car. Make sure to adjust the car seat so that your body will be relaxed and not stiff. Since you are travelling by land, you should take as many road stops as you can so that you can go out and stretch a bit. This way, your joints and muscles won't be stiff. Taking road stops, however, will extend your travel time. Nevertheless, you have the luxury of stretching o By plane. If you want to get to your destination fast, then by air is the best way to go. You will have less time of discomfort compared to long drives. You still need to walk around and stretch, as permitted on the plane, so that your joints won't get stiff. You can do some knee-leg extensions, ankle rotations, or neck rolls during the travel time.

o By boat. This may be the most relaxed mode of travel you can opt for, and also the most scenic. However, you will be exposed to changes in the temperature which can also trigger flare ups. Make sure that you pack clothes accordingly so that you can adjust to temperature changes with ease.

o By bus or train. Similar to air travel, there may be constraints in space when you travel by bus or train. As much as it is permitted, try to stand up and stretch or move around. If not, you can do knee-leg extensions, ankle rotations, or neck rolls during the travel time.

Different kinds of transportation pose different challenges for people with psoriatic arthritis. Make sure you consider the comfort level as you decide on the best way to travel.

When you get to your destination, do not forget to enjoy yourself. Usually, people travel to go on vacations, but even if you are travelling for work, it doesn't mean that you should be all stressed and worried. Take the time to relax. While on travel, make sure that you still eat healthy foods, maintain a good posture, be careful with how you carry things, get enough rest, drink plenty of water and take medications as necessary.

Living with Someone who has Psoriatic Arthritis

People with psoriatic arthritis will tell you that it is hard to live with them. They are in pain most of the time, which can make them irritable, cranky and moody. They can easily change plans and can be quite unpredictable. Their abilities may always be affected depending on the symptom that is triggered. People who live with them will often find themselves asking, "How can I help you?" They may get an answer sometimes, but often they won't get anything. Not many people who suffer from psoriatic arthritis will easily accept help from others. They will want a semblance of independence and will feel embarrassed to ask for or receive help. But even if they say otherwise, they do need help. If you reach out or deep down into the mind and emotions of someone dealing with psoriatic arthritis, here is how you they need help and how you can be a better influence for them:

1. "If you see me struggling, help me."

   Those with psoriatic arthritis will have stiff joints or swollen joints and they will be in constant pain. They will have a loose grip and may have difficulty holding things, especially opening bottles. So if you see them struggling to get a bottle open, or getting a drink, don't be ashamed to help them open it. It will make a difference in their life.

2. You can ask them about their pain.

   They may naturally not want to talk about it, but they really do want to get it out of their chest. The discomfort, the anguish and the feeling of helplessness can be overwhelming for them and getting to talk about it is one way of relaxing. Whether they answer you or not, make sure to ask your loved one how they are feeling. Just the fact that you care enough to inquire of their pain will make them feel better. They may not always look sick, but they can feel it. They won't forget how the pain feels like even if they are not suffering from a flare up. Similarly, when they are experiencing a good day, do your best to help them enjoy moments when they are not in pain. When you talk to them, make sure that you use uplifting, encouraging words. Sometimes, even just planning for an activity or a vacation can ease the feelings of loneliness and helplessness. It is important that you do not show fake interest or roll your eyes whenever they talk about their treatment plans or a new symptom they are feeling.

This can happen when you already know so much about their condition and you have lived with them for so long. Do not be tired about asking them. They need you to ask them. They need you to care. They need someone they can talk to about their condition. They may seem simple or repetitive to you but they mean a great deal to those who have the condition. It is not easy for them but even a simple, "How are you today?" can bring such great comfort.

3. Allow them to move at their own pace.

    So they will wake up slowly, or lay in bed a little while longer. They may move slower than you, even talk more slowly. It is not because they are lazy. It is because they are in pain. The joints are either swollen or stiff. They can't move around too much. They ache all over. For this reason, they will move agonizingly slow and can even be cranky. Let them move at their own pace, do not ever rush them as if they are deliberately slowing own to irritate you. Moving is a huge thing for them, especially during flare ups.

4. Don't minimize their pain.

   You may have been around someone with psoriatic arthritis for so long that you have been used to their flare ups. Here's a gentle reminder—the pain is unbearable for them and the symptoms worsen over time. Do not ever think that they are just acting up, or the symptoms are just the same and they are simply overreacting. Instead, help the patient go through the symptoms, then encourage them to check with their doctors regularly so that adjustments in their medication or therapies can be made and the pain can be reduced. It is like saying to a very sad or frustrated child to simply stop crying—it never works that way. Be the one that ends a helping hand and a listening ear.

5. Support them in making good purchases.

   This means that you guide and offer financial or moral support to them s they make choices on buying the things that will make their life easier, such as good shoes, good pillows, maybe even a wheelchair.

People with psoriatic arthritis don't naturally go on buying things that are helpful for them. They often deny themselves and put off purchasing things that can really be helpful. Simple things like lightweight mugs, lightweight sweepers, lightweight luggage, and even electronic can openers can help them a great deal. Encourage them to make these purchases as it will be good for them in the long run. It's not about the money but the comfort. If you can buy it for them, all the better. This action will show them how much you really care.

6. Don't forget that psoriatic arthritis is chronic. Psoriatic arthritis is lingering and progressive. There will be days when your loved one will feel better and appear like there is nothing wrong. There will be days when they are in so much pain. Celebrate the good days but do not forget all about their condition. There is no easy fix to this persistent disease. You don't have to make them forget, you just need to help them manage it. It is good if you can pay attention to the

triggers whenever you are together. This way, you can help them identify the cues of the onset of a symptom and do the appropriate action like take medication. It is good if you can learn when they are in pain or they are trying to hide it. Naturally, they won't just cry out or scream when they are in pain because they don't want to draw unwanted attention, even if it's from you. Helping them excuse from a social situation by not making mention of their condition is a BIG deal. No patient wants to be always reminded that they have psoriatic arthritis, nor do they want to shout it out to the whole world.

7. During flare days be ready.

The people with psoriatic arthritis that you live with will suffer most when they are most fatigued. They will also be most irritable at those times. So even if they are cranky with you, make sure that you can get their heating pad or ice pack ready. Both should be available because you are not sure what kind of flare up is going to happen. Always check and make sure that your freezer has an ice pack and that a heating pad is readily accessible. Even if you are not in the house, your patient can readily access the needed materials that can help soothe their pain. They may forget to return it to the right pace, but you can do it for them, so the next time there is an attack, the items are still there and can be easily accessed for use.

8. Checking on your patient frequently is not bad. Patients can easily slip into a state of depression or helplessness. After an attack, they may just succumb to fatigue and stay holed up in their beds. This can lead them to feel even worse about themselves. It is a good time to check on them and talk, even just to make sure that they are doing well.

9. Help them exercise and deal with stress. Sometimes, even the simplest of stretching exercises can be difficult for patients with psoriatic arthritis. As much as you can, you can help your loved one exercise and get mobile. Be their exercise

accountability partner. Too little activity is bad as it can cause stiffness. Too much activity, on the other hand, can cause pain. Walk with them, go swimming or cycling. Be lie their therapist when it comes to reminding them to exercise. Remind them of the importance of moving and staying active. You can also be the one that can help them manage their stress levels. Help them identify things and situations that trigger their stress and guide them through stress reduction techniques such as meditation, yoga, prayer and others. Help them avoid anxiety triggers so that they won't feel frazzled and trigger an inflammation attack. For example, they will be anxious in the morning when they have to prepare their lunch packs, you don't have to always prepare it for them, you can encourage them to prepare it in the evening.

10. Help them eat healthy and maintain a good weight. When the patient has been suffering from psoriatic arthritis for a long time, they won't have enough motivation to eat healthy. They may even think

"what's the use of eating healthy when I suffer anyway. Might as well enjoy all the foods that I can." Remind them that the more they eat unhealthily, the greater the risk for triggering inflammation and flare ups. They may not have the necessary motivation to keep their ideal weight and eat the ideal foods, but you can help them in this regard. Remind them of the risks of obesity and too much weight on their joints. When they carry extra weight, they will hurt their knees, ankles, feet and hips. They will also be more fatigued and lack energy. With your voice reminding them, they will be more aware of the need to keep an ideal weight.

To help them eat healthy, make sure that you keep only healthy foods in the house. Do not tempt them to eat junk foods just because you like junk foods and keep them in the pantry. You are their best help for controlling their appetites and urges. Don't skip meals so they don't skip meals, too. Not only do you help them, you will also benefit from the set-up as you will require yourself to eat healthy and maintain your own ideal weight. It's a win-win situation.

11. Don't skimp on sleep.

Everyone needs to have enough hours of sleep, regardless of whether you are healthy or you are suffering from psoriatic arthritis. Lack of sleep brings fatigue and chronic fatigue is common for patients who have psoriatic arthritis. It's often even more trying than the inflammation. When they lack energy and are easily tired, their moods and their quality of life are also greatly affected. Make sure you advise your patient to get enough sleep. To help them, you should also sleep early. Dim lights, good temperature and even essential oils can help both of you get a restful sleep. Stay away from alcohol and caffeine — not only are these inflammatory foods, they also keep the sleepiness away. When there are times that the patient cannot get a good night's rest, make sure that he gets to take naps during the day to energize him.

12. Get a support system.

   This will work both ways. You should get your patient a support system of family members, friends, a therapist, or a support group of those who have the same condition or have overcome the condition. This will help them deal with psoriatic arthritis better. Similarly, you may also need a support system. It won't be easy caring for and living with someone who has psoriatic arthritis. It can take a toll on your physical, mental and emotional well-being as well. Depending on the severity of their condition, you may have to get your patient assistive care. ON the other hand, you may also need to go out with other friends so you can talk about how you are coping, what you are feeling or to just relax yourself, so that when you go back to caring for your patient, you are refilled with motivation and inspiration.

13. Watch out for problems other than the symptoms

   Psoriatic arthritis and its symptoms can just be the tip of the iceberg. Your loved one can be suffering from other conditions and you need to be watchful. Cardiovascular disease, diabetes and other mental health problems can arise as the disease progresses. Monitor their symptoms and be on the lookout for new ones. If you can go to their doctor's check up with them, it will be good so that you can hear the things he discusses as well as mention things that your patient may forget. Sometimes, increased urination, chest pain, and unusual fatigue are not just aggravated symptoms of psoriatic arthritis but can be the beginning signs of diabetes or heart problems. Better safe than sorry. Early intervention can save lives.

14. Continue to be educated.

As they say, knowledge is power. It really is. The more you know about psoriatic arthritis, the more you can care for your patient regarding his symptoms and needs. As you gain knowledge of how it affects your patient, you will get a better idea of how you can help them go through a flare, and you can have better control of your emotions. There are so much information you can find about psoriatic arthritis from books, forums, and support groups. You can check out for new and better treatments that come up, latest news and tips for managing psoriatic arthritis. Remember, medical research is ongoing and there will always be something new to know and apply in terms of nutrition, exercises, therapy, and pain reduction methods.

15. Don't ever give up.

It will be easy to just give up especially when you have a patient that has suffered psoriatic arthritis for years. It is easy for them to just accept their fate. And it can be just as easy for you to give up on finding the best possible treatment. Don't! Just because the first treatments don't work doesn't mean that you cannot offer your patient the relief he deserves. When initial medication isn't working, go back to the doctor to get new ones. When a therapy isn't easing the symptoms, maybe the patient needs a different kind. You can go see a different rheumatologist if you are not satisfied with the progress of the relief. There is always hope and there is always a better option available. Don't lose hope and don't succumb to the fears of the disease.

You can't allow psoriatic arthritis to take over your patient's life, and certainly not yours. Your lives don't have to revolve around the sickness but carrying the burden together will make life easier for you. Find out stuff that you can do and do it with all your heart. There is nothing more beautiful that people caring for each other. Not everyone can cope the same way, each individual is unique. Who would know better how to help the person you live with than you? While psoriatic arthritis can be challenging, you can both adopt ways to make life not just bearable, but also meaningful.

Chapter Seven: Get Some Motivation

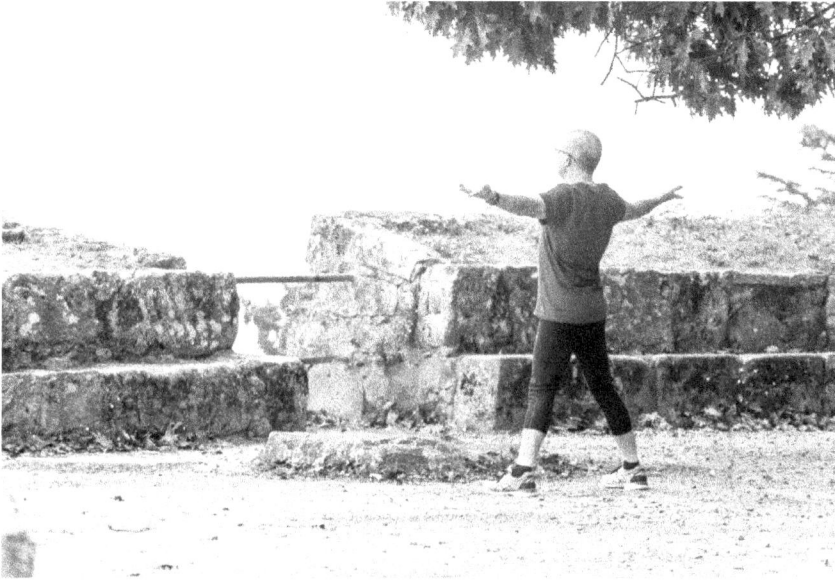

Severe pain, stiff joint, and swelling different parts of the body are some of the debilitating symptoms that patients with psoriatic arthritis suffer. Along with these physical pains can come mental issues like loneliness, despair, feelings of helplessness and depression. With the physical pain they go through, they don't naturally have a good outlook in life. They can not only be cranky, but also gloomy. How can they think about being productive, least of all happy? They face a life that is promised with so much pain, pain that will not go away until the day they die. How can they even think pleasant thoughts?

Well, if you are someone who has psoriatic arthritis or you live with someone who does, you shouldn't have to think that way. Success is never out of reach, whether you have just been diagnosed or you have been suffering for years. In this chapter, you will discover stories about people who have suffered through years and years of symptoms of psoriatic arthritis and yet led successful, productive lives.

Yes, you are not alone! There are many people out there who have the same fate as you, but they did not succumb to loneliness or despair. Instead they rose above their situations and serve as a beacon of light to those who suffer the same condition. There is a chance to live a more meaningful life, and it is something you can grasp. Allow the stories to inspire you, even though you don't have psoriatic arthritis, and let their strategies motivate you to stay physically and mentally strong!

Prominent People with Psoriatic Arthritis

Phil Mickelson

One of the most famous persons with psoriatic arthritis is pro-golfer Phil Mickelson. He shares that he experienced mysterious pain during the 2012 US Open. He found it hard to walk as there was excruciating pain near his right ankle. After this, he had pain in his fingers and wrist. He would then think that his pain came as a result of his rigorous training for the sport. But he didn't do anything to injure himself. In the beginning, the pain passed. However, in the weeks leading up to the US Open, the pain spread from the localized areas and became more severe.

Two days before the tournament started, he was in agonizing pain. He could not even get out of his bed. This time, he did not just chalk it up to training and slowed down. Instead, he went to a doctor and sought professional help. He was diagnosed by a rheumatologist with psoriatic arthritis and was given anti-inflammatory medications to alleviate his pain. He still played in the tournament and got fourth place. It was not easy for him, as golf was his life.

Nevertheless, he did not sulk about it or kept it under wraps. Instead, he helped raise awareness for the disease because he believes that early diagnosis and early treatment can help people. He set up a website that discusses the disease and how crucial it is for patients to get help as soon as they can. There is information on different risk factors for psoriatic arthritis, symptoms as well as possible treatments. His website is co-sponsored by the National Psoriasis Foundation and the Arthritis Foundation.

Mickelson tried a variety of medications like nonsteroidal anti-inflammatory drugs (NSAIDs), disease modifying antirheumatic drugs (DMARDs) and biologics as the tumor necrosis factor (TNF) inhibitor. With the right care, medication and the support of his family, Mickelson got back on the golf course. His pain was reduced and the disability was prevented. Today, his arthritis is under control. Treatment and management is an ongoing process and the same has been true for this superstar. In 2013, he became the British Open champion. He did not allow his ailment to get the better of him. He overcame it with the right means and the right attitude.

He is not just an overcomer, he is also an influencer. He is using his celebrity status to motivate people that there is life even with psoriatic arthritis. He has been in the professional golf arena for many years now because he allowed himself to get an early diagnosis and corresponding treatment. He did not let the stigma of it cause him to draw back and be depressed about his situation. He is now a vocal advocate of psoriatic arthritis and other kinds of arthritis, constantly reminding his audience that even though arthritis can be present for the rest of his life, it doesn't mean he can't enjoy his life.

There will be times when he will have good days; there will be times he will be in pain. But he believes, and he encourages many people, to not lose hope and to rise above their situation by finding the most appropriate pain management plan and enjoying as much of life as they can. Phil Mickelson is an inspiration—he is still playing golf and winning tournaments, despite his condition.

Shawn Lane

A musician's best assets are their hands and ears. When you are a guitarist and you have arthritis, it can seriously wreak havoc in your mind, not to mention your physical body. Shawn Lane is a famed guitarist and is respected as one of the greatest of all time. When he was 13 years old, he was diagnosed with a severe case of psoriatic arthritis. The symptoms were so severe that he would spend days in his bed, writhing in pain. However, with the right medication and therapy, he was able to play with a band called the Black Old Arkansas and became quite popular.

Despite his condition, and the pain that he suffers during flare ups, he was able to make great music and play the lead guitar role. Shawn Lane had the opportunity to work with many popular musicians. His life is an inspiration not just to artists but also simple people, especially the youth. You don't have to be limited by your condition, his life speaks. Where there is talent, there is opportunity, and you need to make the most out of this opportunity. Shawn Lane died of pulmonary fibrosis in 2003. People diagnosed with psoriatic arthritis can have a scarring of the lung tissues as well. A life well lived is an inspiration to al. If you have psoriatic arthritis, think of Shawn Lane and be motivated to go through life's challenges the way he had. Movement using his fingers and writs may have be difficult and painful but his love for music overshadowed this pain and caused him to break through and make a name for himself all over the world.

Byron Janis

A pianist needs his fingers to make beautiful music. But what happens to a pianist when his fingers are afflicted with psoriatic arthritis? This is the problem that child prodigy Byron Janis faced back in 1973. He would be in so much pain as he practiced playing his keys, yet he did not give up. Since age 4, he had been a piano star, a protégé of the world-renowned Vladimir Horowitz. He continued to pay the piano. No one knew that he was suffering from debilitating effects of psoriatic arthritis because he altered his playing style and just continued to make music. During that time he was diagnosed, arthritis was quite looked down upon, much more psoriatic arthritis. This is the reason that he did not publicly disclose his condition until 1985. There was a social stigma that came with pain and he did not want people to feel pity for him. He just continued to play and make beautiful music. At a concert in the White House in 1985, however, he felt that he had to disclose his condition, not to gain pity or kindness from the public, but to be a voice of inspiration. Byron Janis proudly announced that he may have arthritis but "arthritis does not have me". What a powerful statement of positivity! He may have been suffering, but the suffering won't limit him. He may have pain, but pain won't dictate how he lives his life. And he will live his life to the fullest and inspire many people with his music, albeit it may be painstaking to achieve.

He became the ambassador for the arts of the Arthritis Foundation. Janis has tried both traditional pharmacological as well as alternative means for managing psoriatic arthritis. His autobiography declares how he understands that arthritis may not be good for pianists, but playing the piano is good for arthritis. He never stopped playing the piano, crediting the exercise as good for his aching hands. He also acknowledges that his deep spiritual beliefs have helped him get through his condition and live a meaningful life. His love for music also was a fuel for his passion for life. Indeed, nothing is impossible in life, especially if you have a good outlook. Perspective can mean everything. Arthritis cannot lay hold of your life; it doesn't have to be the chain that binds you. You can overcome it and live life the way you want to.

Bob Murphy

Another pro golfer that suffered from psoriatic arthritis is sportscaster Bob Murphy. His battle with psoriatic arthritis started when he was 43 years old. He had been a pro golfer since 1968 and he started to feel the pain of the inflammation in 1986. He had been in so much pain that in 1987, he could not pay golf anymore. He had a difficult time holding a golf club, much less swinging it. In his interview with the National Psoriasis Foundation, he tells the story of how six of his ten fingers became swollen, stiff and disfigured. The skin on his legs was covered with red scales. After a check-up with a rheumatologist, he was diagnosed with psoriasis and psoriatic arthritis. Because he was diagnosed early and correctly, he received medication and treatments that included magnet therapy.

He was able to overcome psoriatic arthritis and went back to playing golf. He even won eleven more times during the Champion Tour that was held for senior pro golfers. You may get diagnosed with psoriatic arthritis early on in life or in your later years, but the symptoms and the pain will always be the same—they are debilitating and can ruin your life if you let it. But look at Bob Murphy. What he did was not wallow win self-pity or just cry out in pain. He got treatment until he was able to manage his condition.

More than that, he went back to what he loves to do best—golf—and he even won championships despite his condition. He is a perfect example of a person who does not give up on his dreams. He was already in his 40s when he was diagnosed and started suffering through psoriatic arthritis. He could have just given up on life, stayed home and nurtured himself. But he chose to fight back and reclaim his life because he believes that there is more for him. Life won't end when you have psoriatic arthritis. It can even be just the beginning of your developing into a stronger character.

Dennis Potter

Dennis Potter is a famed British dramatist who suffered from psoriatic arthritis. He died in 1994 from psoriatic atropathy, a severe case of the arthritis. He was in and out of hospitals, but even though he suffered from the arthritis, he still continued to write dramas. In one of his dramas he made a character named Philip Marlow, who died of the same condition he suffered with. He wanted people to realize the gravity of the situation Potter's hands were whittled on to clubs as they deformed through time, that he had to tape a pen to his fist in order to write. Even though it was hard when his hands were clenched permanently, he did not give up on his love for writing and producing great stories. You, too, don't have to give up on the things you love.

You can continue writing, working, cooking, whatever it is you like doing. The pain may become unbearable at times, but you need to persevere. Make sure to get the right treatment so that you can stop the progression of the disease and still enjoy your life. You can be in control of your health, especially if you have a good support system.

Seamus Mullen

Seamus Mullen is an award-winning restaurateur, excellent chef and author. When he was first diagnosed with arthritis in 2007, he experienced chronic pain all over his body. He felt that life will never be the same again. He advises people that they need to know that they are not alone. There are people all over the world suffering from the same conditions and they can educate themselves about the disease so that they can have a better understanding of what they are going through. You don't always have to depend on the medical community for answers. You can join support groups where you can get together and talk about how you are feeling, how you see life, what changes you can make, how others were able to overcome, and most especially to be encouraged. Mullen still undergoes treatment and medication, but the best help he has received in overcoming this condition is the support from the community that surrounds him with hope.

The Ordinary Joe

Then there is the story of the ordinary Joe. The average worker, the simple family man, the working mother, and the young student. All of whom suffer pain in their joints, swelling in their knees or elbows. They can't move their neck or raise their arms without pain. They find it hard to get up in the morning or to even sleep at night. The pain wracks throughout their whole body. Moving around has become such a tremendously difficult task.

Relationships are affected simply because those who suffer from psoriatic arthritis can be quite moody especially when they are in pain. It can be hard to understand and be patient with their mood swings much more with their anger in life. Of course, they question why it had to happen to them. They were too young, too rich, too beautiful, too ambitious. There is so much of life ahead of them only to be challenged by this dreaded disease. But wait—they do not lose hope. They move on despite the pain. Even with swollen fingers, mothers continue to care for their children, to cook and do the laundry, to clean the house and give them baths. Even when there is pain in the neck and back, the father of four continue to go to work every day so that he can put food on the table and send his kids to school.

Despite always feeling exhausted because of flare ups, the diligent student continues to go to his classes and do his homework because he dreams of becoming a doctor who will one day find the cure for psoriatic arthritis. These people, ordinary men and women, do not give up on life just because of the debilitating pain. When they have bad days, they may cry and become sad. But the have hope, especially during the good days when there is no pain. They know that they cannot give up on life because they have a family, they have dreams, and they have goals.

Understand this; you don't have to find a celebrity story in order to be inspired. All across the globe there are hundreds of thousands of people who have psoriatic arthritis and these people continue to live their lives normally. They go to work, go to school, take care of families or businesses, play sports and do various arts, in spite of the pain they go through every day and in spite of the knowledge that they will go through this for the rest of their life. Not everyone who is diagnosed with psoriatic arthritis cave in to the loneliness and pain, not all of them suffer from mental illnesses because of the exhaustion they feel. In fact, most of them are strong. If they can go through the physical pain that comes and goes and attacks without warning, they can be strong in mind as well and overcome.

You can be that ordinary Joe. You can be that simple Jane. Suffering from pain and unbearable discomfort and yet strong in your resolve to live a full life. Don't be afraid to do the things you are passionate about. Don't be afraid to travel, do new things or go on great adventures. You just need to start by getting the right diagnosis and the right treatment or management plan. If you have experienced the symptoms, don't be anxious about going to go to a doctor.

Don't be scared to join a support group. Don't be embarrassed to ask for help. It could spell a big difference in your life. If you hold back, it may be too late for you. So, as with the people mentioned in the stories in this chapter, go and pursue that treatment even as you continue living the life that you have always dreamed of. And do not let go until the end.

It Can Happen to Anyone

Psoriatic arthritis can happen to anyone. You can be young or old, rich or poor, a virtual unknown or a high-profile celebrity. The symptoms can affect everyone the same way, but how you deal with it doesn't have to be a cookie cutter reaction. Where other people can limit themselves to a life of pain, you can overcome. You can be better. You can live more. May you be inspired by the stories found in this chapter so you will have a better perspective in life and a brighter outlook for the future.

What's more, may your life be a shining beacon and a great testimony of hope that in spite of having psoriatic arthritis, which can last the rest of your life, you can have a meaningful, full, happy life.

The key is to have a good perspective in life. Keep yourself motivated. Who knows, the next book about psoriatic arthritis can be the testimony of your powerful, successful life. You can be the next ambassador or advocate of arthritis, inspiring people to overcome their condition and the pain that threatens to consume their life. Wouldn't that be something to look forward to?

Conclusion

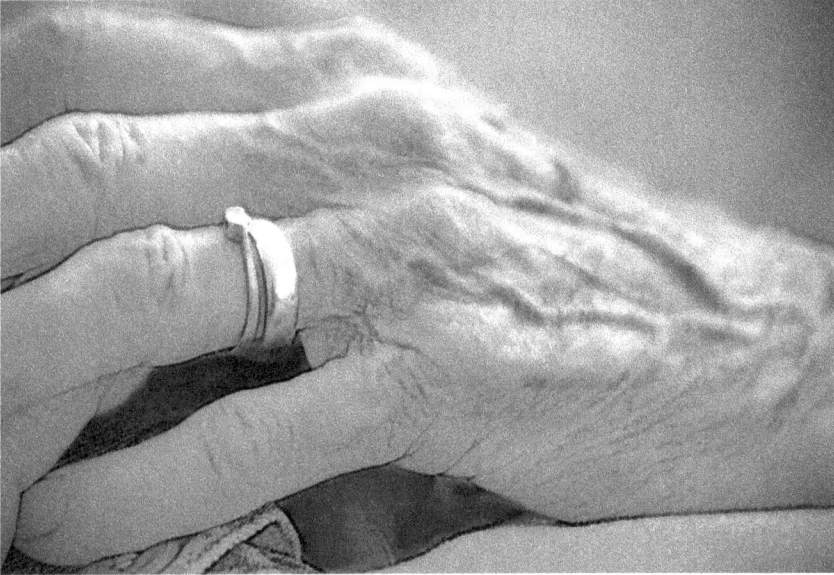

First of all, if you haven't been diagnosed with psoriatic arthritis and you experience any or some of the symptoms outlined in this book, you need to go to a doctor and get the proper diagnosis. Only then can you decide on the best treatment plan you will undertake. It is important to remember that early diagnosis can lead to early treatment. When there is intervention at the early stages of psoriatic arthritis, you can stop the progress of this degenerative disease.

Whatever your age, race, gender or status in life, if you have been diagnosed with psoriatic arthritis, it can be the biggest challenge you will ever face in life. You may be overcome with the physical pain caused by the swelling, stiffness and inflammation. You will also be affected mentally and emotionally. Psoriatic arthritis, being incurable, will last for the rest of your life—and you have to live with it.

That's right. You have to live with it. Now the choice you need to make is how you will live with it. You can choose to be sad over your seeming misfortune and just withdraw from life. Or you can continue living your daily life without much hope of getting better. Or you can live to overcome and make the most of your life, pursue your passions and achieve your goals in spite of what you feel. In the beginning, the biggest question you will answer will be what are the things you can do and the things you can't do anymore. As you accept your condition, you will be faced with certain limitations. But these limitations should not spell the end of your happiness and success in life. There are so many things you can do to not only curb the effects of psoriatic disease in your life, but to also give you the power to live more effectively and develop meaningful relationships. You can go for therapy, take medication, proceed with alternative treatments—there are so many options available for you.

The most important thing is to remember that in spite of having psoriatic arthritis, your attitude towards your condition is your choice and your choice alone. You can have the best doctor in the world, access to the best medical treatments and the best support group ever, but if your attitude sucks, you won't get the best out of it. How you respond to the pain you feel and the management plans set in place will largely affect the quality of your life.

Understand that there will be bad days and there will be good days, and you need to practice a lot of patience and perseverance. From the moment of diagnosis to the rest of your life, you will have to stay strong and positive, especially during the challenging days of pain.

Remember, a bad day does not equate to a bad life. Just because you have psoriatic arthritis means that you have a bad life. Because it is chronic, bad days will be just around the corner. But as some of the famous celebrities who battled through psoriatic arthritis said, you may have arthritis, but you shouldn't let it have you! You can be your own positive voice.

You can be your own advocate. Write down some high quality goals in life you want to achieve and in all earnest, enjoy life and achieve those goals. You can do it! Especially if you remember that you are not alone. You don't have to feel awful about your condition. You can rise about it. It's not enough to simply, you can choose to thrive. You can be successful. There is more to life for you. The world is waiting for you to share your story of life!

Photo Credits

References

Psoriatic Arthritis – EmedicineHealth.com

https://www.emedicinehealth.com/psoriatic_arthritis/article_em.htm#psoriatic_arthritis_pictures

Alternative Treatments for Psoriatic Arthritis – EverydayHealth.com

https://www.everydayhealth.com/arthritis/psoriatic-arthritis/alternative-treatments-psoriatic-arthritis/

Psoriatic Arthritis: 9 Natural Remedies – Health.com

https://www.health.com/health/gallery/0,,20516045,00.html#traditional-chinese-medicine-0

Best Natural Remedies for Psoriatic Arthritis – Healthline.com

https://www.healthline.com/health/psoriatic-arthritis/natural-remedies#7

Psoriatic Arthritis – MedicineNet.com

https://www.medicinenet.com/psoriatic_arthritis/article.htm #what_does_the_future_hold_for_patients_with_psoriatic_ar thritis

Psoriatic Arthritis - Can Homeopathy Help Treat it? – Lybrate.com

https://www.lybrate.com/topic/psoriatic-arthritis-can-homeopathy-help-treat-it/9c963d24f9f2cadc93ec86b9e592c7ae

9 Foods to Eat or Avoid for Psoriatic Arthritis - EverydayHealth.com

https://www.everydayhealth.com/hs/psoriatic-arthritis-management-treatment/psoriatic-arthritis-foods/

Psoriatic Arthritis: Overview – MayoClinic.org

https://www.mayoclinic.org/diseases-conditions/psoriatic-arthritis/symptoms-causes/syc-20354076

Psoriatic Arthritis - Rheumatology.org

https://www.rheumatology.org/I-Am-A/Patient-Caregiver/Diseases-Conditions/Psoriatic-Arthritis

Psoriatic Arthritis – Medscape.com

https://emedicine.medscape.com/article/2196539-overview

Psoriatic Arthritis – Rheumatology.org

https://www.rheumatology.org/I-Am-A/Patient-Caregiver/Diseases-Conditions/Psoriatic-Arthritis

How to Manage Psoriatic Arthritis without Drugs – WebMD.com

https://www.webmd.com/arthritis/psoriatic-arthritis/psoriatic-arthritis-nondrug-treatment

Best Natural Remedies for Psoriatic Arthritis – HealthLine.com

https://www.healthline.com/health/psoriatic-arthritis/natural-remedies

www.ingramcontent.com/pod-product-compliance
Lightning Source LLC
Chambersburg PA
CBHW072234290326
41934CB00008BA/1285